Grandma's Natural Remedies and Ancient Herbal Recipes Volume 8

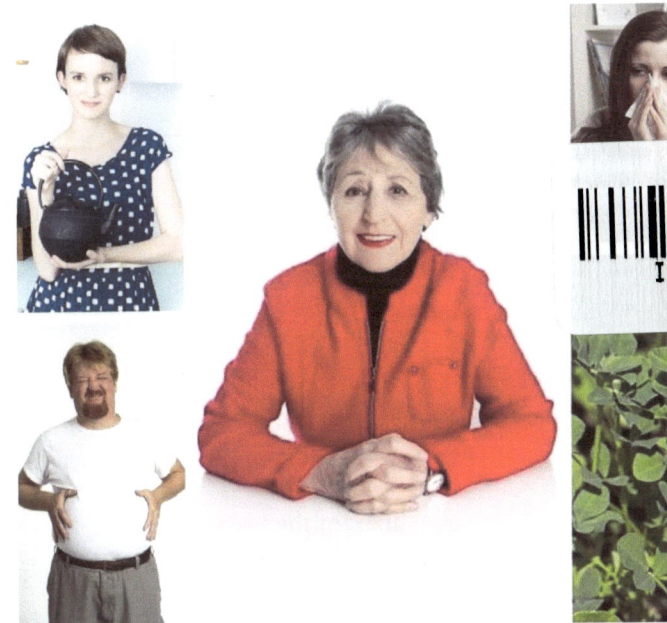
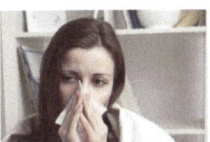

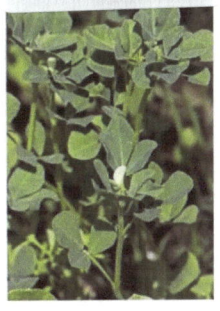

Dueep Jyot Singh

Natural Remedy Series

Mendon Cottage Books

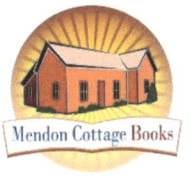

JD-Biz Publishing

Disclaimer

The information is this book is provided for informational purposes only. It is not intended to be used and medical advice or a substitute for proper medical treatment by a qualified health care provider. The information is believed to be accurate as presented based on research by the author.

The contents have not been evaluated by the U.S. Food and Drug Administration or any other Government or Health Organization and the contents in this book are not to be used to treat cure or prevent disease.

The author or publisher is not responsible for the use or safety of any diet, procedure or treatment mentioned in this book. The author or publisher is not responsible for errors or omissions that may exist.

Warning

The Book is for informational purposes only and before taking on any diet, treatment or medical procedure, it is recommended to consult with your primary health care provider.

Our books are available at

1. Amazon.com
2. Barnes and Noble
3. Itunes
4. Kobo
5. Smashwords
6. Google Play Books

Table of Contents

Introduction

Grandma was a great believer in natural remedies and cures. She knew that herbs and other plant products, were amazingly efficient, and effective in getting rid of minor ailments, which would be the lot and portion of her large family.

That is why she used all those nostrums, infusions, decoctions, and other herbal products which had been passed on to her by her grandma and so on down the ages. So here is another collection of grandma's natural remedies and ancient herbal recipes to keep you healthy, as well as beautiful.

All these products are easily available right in your garden or in your kitchen. Best of all, they have no aftereffects and they have no side effects. That is because all these products are completely hundred percent natural.

Why are so many people going back to natural remedies and ancient herbal recipes, in the 21st century? That is because they have found that chemical-based drugs and medicines have a short-term effect. They may also come accompanied with toxic effects, and side effects. So you are going to find yourself suffering from these long-term aftereffects. However, that is definitely not the case when you are taking natural remedies, which have been made with hundred percent natural products.

And that is what grandma did. She gathered all the natural products available in her garden, or easily available in the woods, when she went rambling out gathering herbs, and brought them home. These were then used, to cure a number of ailments. Some of them seem rather drastic, but you need to remember that grandma was more of an experimenter. She knew that there was one product in these herbal combinations which did all the magic. The rest were just "filling."

Now how did that happen? How could she not target the exact ingredient which did all the magic, and use just that to cure everybody?

The answer is very simple. Grandma did not learn all her herbal lore from her ancestors. Some of them were learned from the priests, the medicine men, and from her neighbors. Now all of them were rather imbued by their own importance and wanted to make sure that they had a reputation of being very learned among their peers. That is why they added their own bit of mumbo-jumbo to the mixture. So when grandmother went with a sheep to a learned wise man, or medicine man or even a priest, he would roll his eyes and say in thundering tones,

"O woman, the stars are against you. But do not worry, this sheep is going to appease them. Now what you are going to do is you are going to gather the leaves of the sacred basil, when the moon is full tonight. After that, you are going to pick up some ginger, while keeping your head bowed down. Speak to nobody, all this while. Otherwise, the goddess shall get angry with thee. Bring them both home and still keeping quiet, grind them up together and boil them in one glass of water, until half the water has gone back to the heavens. Then feed it to your ailing child to get rid of the fever. Do this for three nights running, and collect enough of these herbs, so that you can feed your child with this magic water twice a day. "

Grandma would naturally be very impressed with such a knowledgeable man's instructions. That is the reason why so many of her herbal remedies collected today and ancient herbal compendiums talk about accompanying chants, full moons, the gatherer dressed in clean white garb at midnight and the rest of showmanship mumbo-jumbo. Nevertheless, it was the basil and the ginger which cured the child off fevers!

So without much resort to loud incantations, here is a collection of grandma's natural remedies and ancient recipes brought to you to help keep you and your family healthy the natural way.

Grandma's Herbal Decoctions

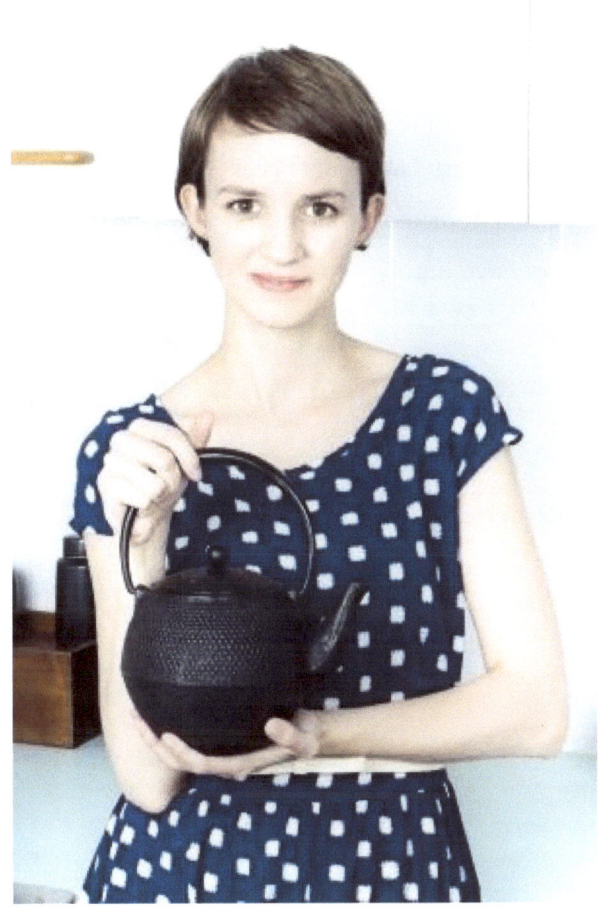

Grandmas decoctions were normally include or infused in a old-fashioned kettle.

Grandma was a great believer in herbal decoctions. This was normally made by putting herbs in water, and then allowing the water to boil till half of it was evaporated. This made sure that all the essence of the herbs was concentrated in that small amount of water. This was extremely powerful, and that was a surefire cure for fevers, coughs, colds, and minor ailments. Sometimes, she added a little bit of molasses to it, in order to make it more palatable, especially when the herbs which were used were extremely bitter. She believed in the theory that the more bitter a herb was, the more powerful it would be in the long run. That is not necessarily true. Nevertheless, grandmother's herbal decoctions were guaranteed effective to get rid of the ailments they were targeting.

Cough/Cold Cure

Now this is a tasty decoction, which is traditionally known as **Kadaa- [kaa dhaa.]** It is not bitter and it is given to children, when they are suffering from Cold and cold related problems in the winter. Adults also love it!

Gather together 2 tablespoons each of fennel seeds, and cumin seeds, four cloves, one inch stick of cinnamon, four Green cardamoms, six peppercorns, 1.5 inches of grated ginger.

Roast all the spices on a griddle, until they give out an aromatic fragrance. Now, grind them all together in a blender. Put 3 cups of water on to boil and add all the spices to it. Once the water has been reduced to half of its original volume, filter it, and drink boiling hot with 1 tablespoon full of honey added to it. Then cover yourself up with warm clothes, and go off to sleep. If you want to add a little bit more of taste, you can always add 3 tablespoons full of milk to this mixture.

I found one of my friends, drinking this kaada instead of tea, in the winter, by just adding the leaves and milk. That is also a good idea. If you do not want to make this again and again, all you have to do is leave it, unstrained, and put it in the fridge. Heat when needed. But grandma made it fresh, and grandma made it hot.

The spices cure you. The ginger gives you warmth. The honey tones up your system. The rest is just for good taste and good health!

Cramps and Joint Pain

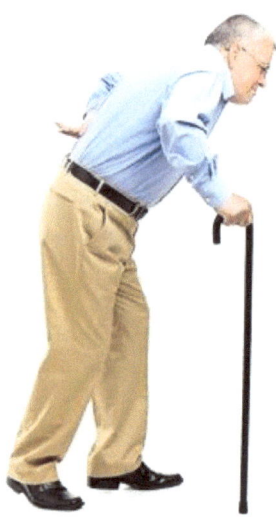

Massage can help in joint pain.

You suffer from joint pain especially when you are a victim of arthritis, gout, or even rheumatism. There are plenty of natural cures in ancient medicine books, and all of them are considered to be effective to get rid of these ailments.

Here are a few of them –

Banana diet

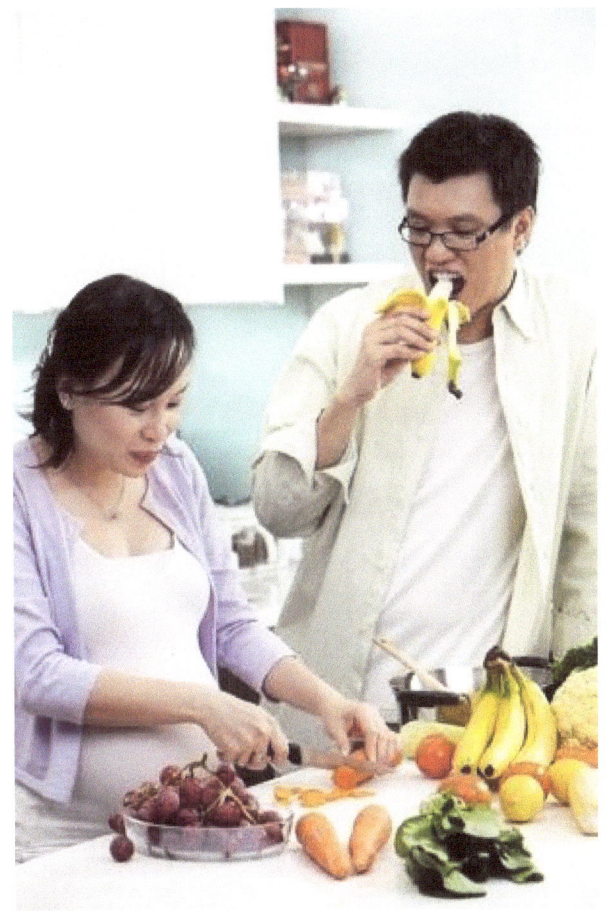

Now this is a remedy told to me by a person suffering from arthritis. He ate only bananas and nothing but bananas for three – four days. In fact, his banana diet went up to anywhere between 9 to 10 bananas per day. He says that he found visible improvement in joint pain.

 Now this much I know, that if you are suffering from cramp in your legs – do you remember just stretching your legs, and then a terrible pain shooting out on your lower leg area and muscles – you can get rid of that permanently by eating two – three bananas for a whole month. Believe it or not, this is a time proven remedy, because the potassium content in the bananas, help cure your muscles. So why should it not cure joint pain?

Neem Remedy

You can also massage the affected areas with neem oil, in case of joint pain.

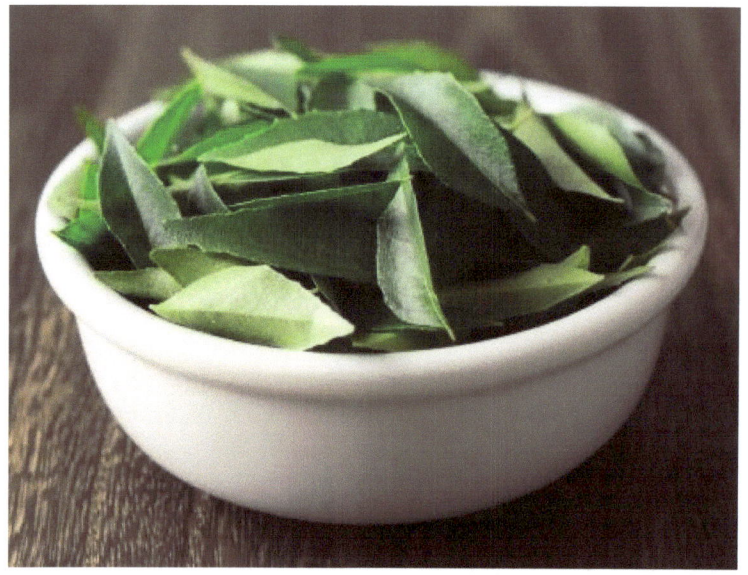

If you have a Neem tree around, just gather some fresh leaves. Grind them with a little bit of water, and strain. Add half a teaspoonful of lemon juice, and drink this once a day, first thing in the morning. If you are suffering from acidity, do not try this remedy. Because Neem is a very powerful herb, this is going to be very bitter, but it is a guaranteed effective cure for pain in your joints.

Lemon Remedy

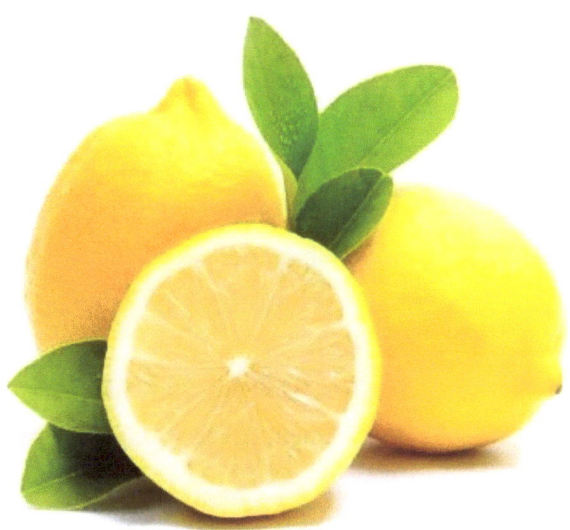

This is for all those people who enjoy eating lots of lemons throughout the year. Squeeze the juice of half a lemon in really hot water. You need to drink that hot water, because that is what is going to cure your joint pain. Drink this at intervals of two hours. That means you are going to have about eight glasses of lemon water, throughout your daily grind.

Do not go by anybody telling you that this is definitely not a good thing for your body, because naturopathy says that people who are suffering from joint problems, and muscle related problems should not eat things that are sour. But lemons do not come under that category here. They may taste sour, but when they are in your body, they are going to act alkaline in nature. Also, the vitamin C is excellent in curing your joint problems.

All right, when I advised this remedy to a person suffering from joint problems, and she drank this juice for two days, she got back to me, ready and ripe for murder.

According to her, the pain had increased. Here is the explanation – It *seems* like it happens that way. That is because of the lemon, trying desperately hard to cure the problem. The pain has not increased, it is just you feeling that it *may have* increased. Because you do not have faith in this cure!

The pain is going to decrease gradually, and within 5 to 7 days, you are going to find a significant improvement. Keep on with this remedy, until you find yourself mobile again.

It is going to be a long-term treatment, but you are curing yourself the natural way aren't you? That is what natural medicine promises you. It promises you that you are going to be cured long-term and permanently. It does not give you airy – fairy promises. So you need to be patient, when you are looking for anything to be cured permanently through natural therapy.

Fenugreek Cure

The East is very used to spices, and that is why fenugreek is an essential part of every spice box here. The leaves are an extremely tasty vegetable and that is why this Greek clover is eaten extensively in the East.

Fenugreek is an extremely good way in which you can get rid of arthritis and rheumatism. Fenugreek leaves should be added to your diet, especially as they are so plentiful in the winter.

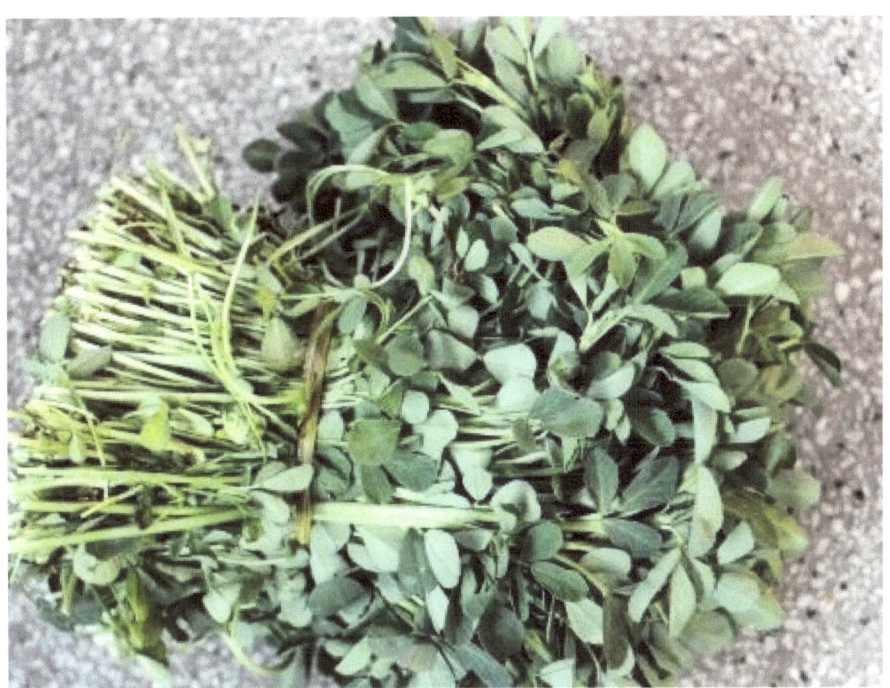

Soak 2 teaspoons of fenugreek seeds in a cup of yogurt. Leave it overnight. If this first thing in the morning. You can do the same thing by soaking them in water and drinking the water in the morning, then chew the fenugreek seeds. Do this every day.

Fenugreek Poultice

Grind some fenugreek seeds in hot water, spread over a piece of cotton cloth and apply on any areas which are suffering from gout. This is going to alleviate any gouty pain.

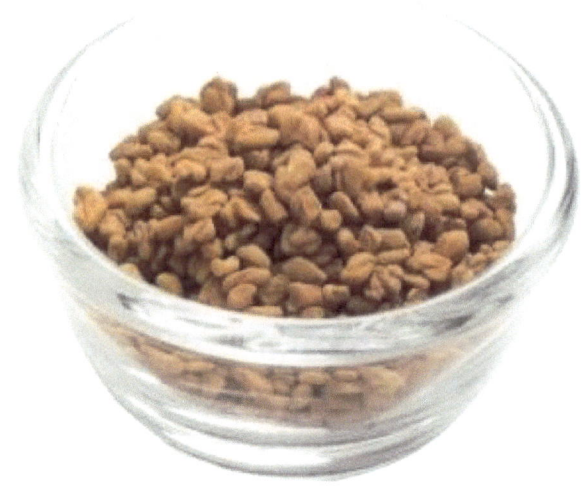

Fenugreek Potato Recipe

Fenugreek is normally eaten traditionally with boiled potatoes and aubergines added. This neutralizes to a great extent the bitter taste of the fenugreek leaves. It is normally used as a contrasting flavor in meat dishes, but I am giving you the vegetable recipe.

Old people in the East are given this dish very often throughout the winter, so that they never suffer from joint pains, or arthritis or even gout.

To make this tasty and healthy dish, you are going to collect –

4 medium-size potatoes, peeled and chopped
One bunch of fresh fenugreek leaves. You also get them frozen, so if you are de – freezing them, use half a packet.

Desi ghee – 2 tablespoons. If you are worried about the cholesterol, use ordinary cooking oil, but it takes half of the fun and flavor out of a tasty delicious dish. You are going to get the way how to make this traditional clarified butter, in the [Appendix](#).

One finely chopped onion

Four cloves of finely chopped garlic

Half a teaspoon each of coriander powder and turmeric powder.

Chili powder and salt to taste. If you want it hot, you can add more chili powder. Try adding rock salt. This is a healthier alternative, and you do not have to worry much about the sodium content. Also, you are not going to get a really salty fenugreek, Ari

One small piece of peeled ginger, grated

One medium-size tomato

Two aubergines, chopped.

There are two ways to prepare this aubergine. One is the traditional way, on which they are roasted on hot charcoals, after oil is applied to their skins. As soon as the skin is burned, it is removed and the flesh added to any dish, to make a thick curry. Or you may just chop them into squares and add them to the dish.

Chop up the fenugreek leaves after washing them. You can either keep the stalks in if you want, or you can remove the stalks. I normally spend half an hour in just removing the leaves, while watching TV, but then, I have plenty of leisure time. That is up to you. After all, fenugreek stalks are also delicious and add to the flavor. But if you are chopping up the stalks, make sure that they are properly chopped into small pieces.

Now place this chopped fenugreek in a bowl, and mix well with salt. You can add a little bit of lemon juice. This is going to neutralize the really bitter taste of the leaves and make it taste milder. Leave this for 20 minutes.

During this time, heat the ghee in a wok and add the garlic, green chilies and onions. Fry on a low heat till the onions are soft and golden brown.

Add the salt and the potatoes, as well as the aubergine flesh or aubergine cubes, and cook, stirring, occasionally for about 10 minutes. You are frying this in a Wok. That means you do not have to add water. Consider this to be stirfried until the potatoes are cooked and soft.

Now add the fenugreek leaves, stir well and allow to cook again. You may want to place the cover on them for a couple of minutes, so that they can cook in their own steam. Add all the spices, and mix well.

There are two ways in which you can add turmeric powder. You can either fry them with the onions in the initial stages of frying, or you can add them along with the vegetables. Both ways should ensure that the turmeric is properly mixed in the dish.

Allow to cook for another five minutes until you think the fenugreek is done. Turn the stove off and add the tomatoes. Mix them together, and let them sit for 10 minutes before serving hot.

I make this tastier by frying the tomatoes on the side on a griddle, while the last stages of cooking of the potato fenugreek is being done. This enhances the tomato flavor.

Get the people suffering from joint problems to eat this delicious and healthy dish at least 3 to 4 times in a week. They are going to find their joint problems improving drastically.

If they think that there is a much of a muchness to the recipe, you can try the same recipe, by replacing the potatoes and aubergines, with pieces of chicken. This is going to give you chicken fenugreek.

Tomato Tip

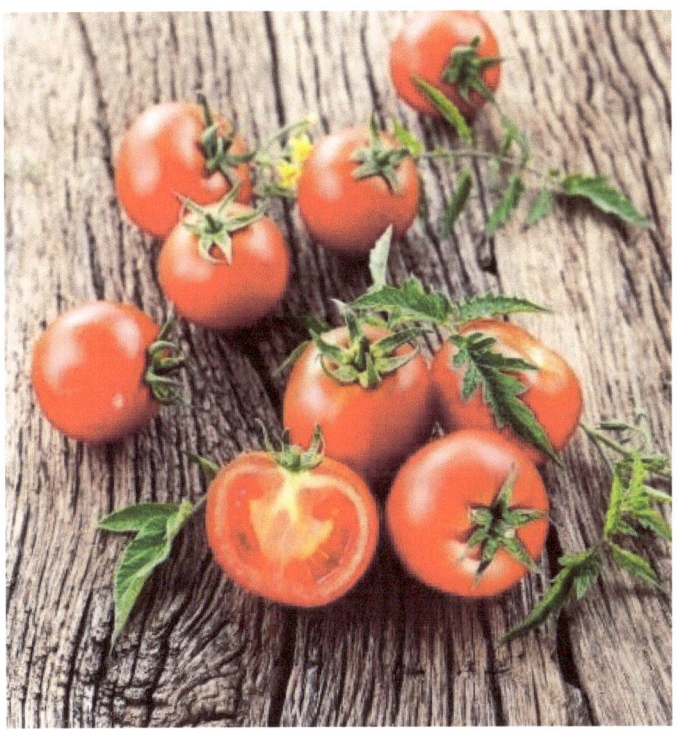

Always remember to seed tomatoes, before you use in cooking. Just use the tomato pulp. This is going to prevent any possible and potential problems related to seeds during digestion.

Here is one cooking tip, which I give to all my friends. Tomato pulp, is best used when you are cooking. Tomato seeds have the tendency of causing trouble, when they get into your tummy, especially if you are suffering from kidney stones.

Some people also say that they aggravate kidney stone problems and then they stop eating tomatoes. Remember tomato pulp, is healthy and nutritious. Just remove the seeds and place them in your garden for organic fertilizer or for growing tomato plants!

Rheumatic Pain

Dried ginger is considered to be quite a good way in which you can get rid of rheumatism. Just take a three piece of dried ginger, and grind it with a marble sized chunk of asafoetida. Now asafoetida is very hot, and so is ginger, so you are going to put them in some milk to make a paste. This is then applied to the affected area giving you pain.

Sit in the sun, so that the ginger as well as the asafoetida, as well as the rays of the sun can heal you.

Massage oil for Rheumatism

I normally make up a massage oil, for people suffering from rheumatism by crushing 3 tablespoons full of powdered nutmeg with three powdered cinnamons and one powdered clove in one cup of sesame oil, or mustard oil. Now, nutmeg, cinnamon and cloves are extremely powerful. So this massage is best done in the winter sun especially when you are sunning yourself. You are going to be surprised to see the positive effects helping cure you.

Do not apply the oil, when it is boiling hot! It should be easy to touch by your massaging hands and bearably warm on the surface of the skin of the affected person.

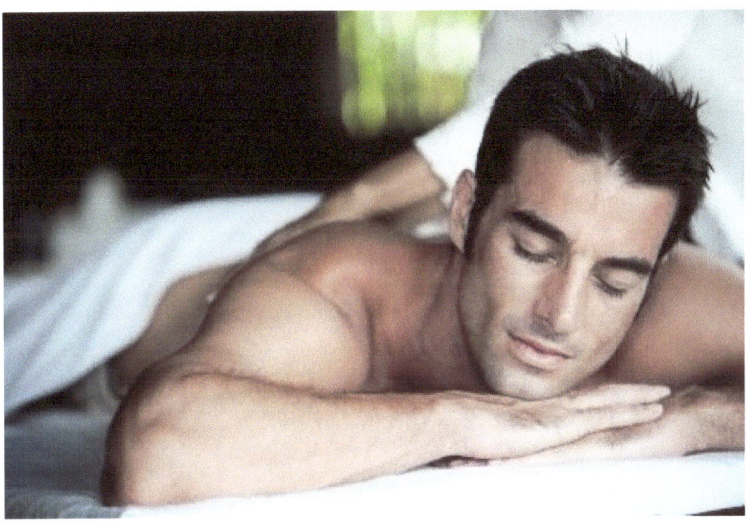

Rheumatism can attack anyone, anywhere. Massaging helps take care of the pain.

Massage this for 10 to 20 minutes, if you have the time. Massage lightly, so that the patient does not feel any pain.

Basil Toothpaste for Keeping Your Teeth Healthy

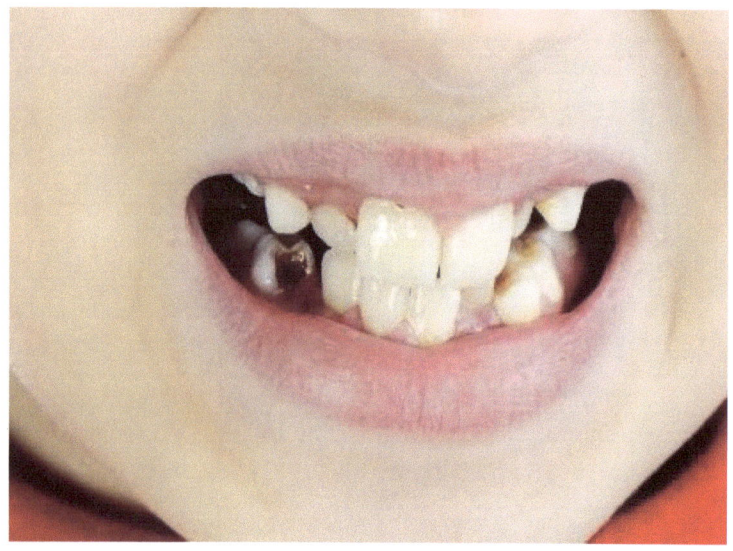

Protect your teeth with natural toothpaste.

Do you have any dried leaves of the sacred basil around? You may find them in your kitchen, if you are using herbs extensively. If you have this basil plant in your garden, well, this is the best way in which you can keep your teeth healthy and you do not have to visit your dentist anymore.

Make up a toothpaste of these products –

2 fistfuls of dried basil – you collect the basil leaves, and then put them out in the shade in a sunny corner of your terrace, covered with a cloth. This is going to protect your drying leaves from dust and insects.

1 tablespoon ground pepper

Three crushed dried cloves

2 teaspoons sea salt

One fistful each of sage and mint leaves.

Juice of one lemon

Half a teaspoon bicarbonate of soda.

Half a pea sized amount of powdered alum, roasted first on the griddle on dry heat.

Three Dried Neem leaves. Why am I adding these neem leaves is that they are among the best natural antiseptics. So I am giving them in this toothpaste, because they are going to heal any potential tooth problems. And the lower number is because they are bitter. If you do not mind a bit of bitter taste, first thing in the morning, and last thing at night, you can increase the amount of neem leaves.

Grind all these ingredients together. Then make a paste of toothpaste consistency with mustard oil. Mix well. Put it in a wide mouthed jar, and place them in your bathroom.

I normally dip the bristle side of my toothbrush in this paste, because I am not squeezing it out of a tube. Then brush your teeth, and say goodbye to any sort of dental problems, pain, cavities, and even bad breath.

Constipation Remedy

Remember that constipation is the bane of all those gourmets, who keep eating rich and indigestible food, without bothering about the consequences. They are also going to suffer from acidity. So the best way to deal with any constipation problems is to change your food habits immediately. Start taking fresh fruits and their juices, a couple of times during the day. Boiled vegetables are good, as well as is milk. Fruits and vegetables with plenty of fibers as well as those with roughage are going to clear up and tone up your system.

Stop eating meat for 2 to 3 days. Add your liquid intake – not tea and coffee, soft drinks or alcoholic beverages – and add to your vegetable and fruit content. Try munching on raw fruit. You are soon going to see your system clearing up really well.

I make sure that I have a 2 L water bottle right next to my bedside before I go to sleep. Because I have the tendency to wake up about three times, every night, I just reach for the bottle, and drink off the water. If you are a healthy sleeper, you would not need to wake up in the night and drink the water before popping off to sleep again. So you are going to finish that water, the first thing in the morning when you are switching off the alarm clock.

You are going to *need* to go to the bathroom within half an hour, thanks to this water, so make sure that you are not rushing off to the office and possibly getting caught in the rush-hour traffic.

This is a traditional constipation remedy, which comes under the heading of Rose jam. It is originally Persian, the land of Rose oil, water, and exotic scents. It is called gul- qand- gool kuh-nd. Literally meaning flower jam.

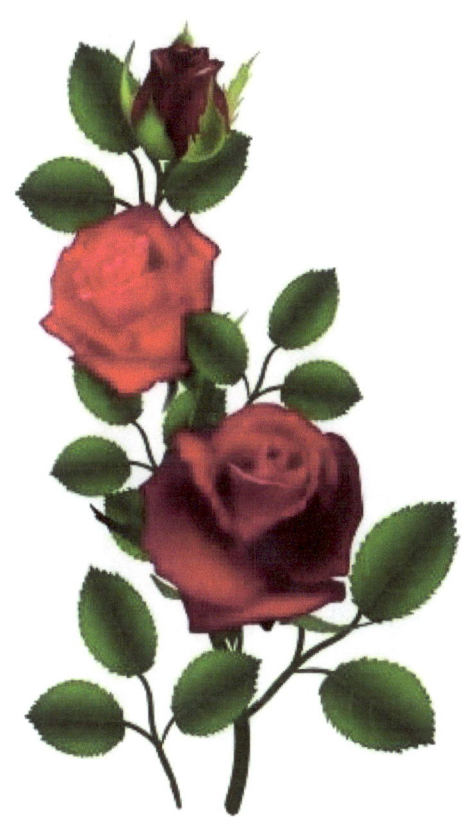

Red roses are best for making this Rose jam.

Gulqand-Rose Jam

This is a traditional Persian recipe, which was brought to the East by the Moguls. You can call it Rose Jam. It is normally used to combat ailments brought about by summer, especially lethargy, sunstroke, exposure to sun, and other conditions related to heat. Also, like I said, this is going to help you, if you are suffering from chronic constipation.

In ancient Ayurveda and in ancient Persian medicine, doctors used to prescribe Gulkand to all those patients suffering from an imbalance in the pulse. Is your summer sweat foul-smelling, especially in the armpit region?

You need a teaspoonful of Gulkand every day with milk at breakfast, lunch and dinner. In the same way, if you are suffering from hemorrhage or nose bleeding, Gulkand will be suggested to you by an eastern medicine man.

The taste is bittersweet and pungent. It is supposed to speed up your metabolism and your digestive system.

In ancient Greek medicine, it was supposed to be a blood purifier making your skin pimple free and without blemishes. Also, if you are suffering from stress and strain, this is an excellent tonic to calm you down.

Hyperacidity is supposedly controlled with Gulkand and also, if you are suffering from constipation, you are going to find your digestive system functioning better with this Rose jam.

The best thing I like about Gulkand is that once it is made, it is going to last for years and years. One of my relatives made it with honey, but I guess that to be overkill. If you have plenty of honey around, you can make it with honey. But that is going to make it even more powerful.

That means you are going to be eating half a teaspoon, three times a day. This antioxidant is a mild laxative, and that is why it will keep your system clear and healthy.

2 ½ tablespoons of Rose jam every morning with hot milk should cure you of chronic constipation.

How to Collect Wild Rose Petals

If you find red rose petals growing in the wild, how lucky you are. This is going to have more percentage of essential oils, especially if you have rosa Damascena around. Somehow, I do not find cultivated rose hybrids to have such a great amount of required essential oils.

Make sure that the rose petals which you collect are pesticide free by washing them thoroughly. Also get rid of the insects and dust. I normally dump them in a bucket full of water, swish them around and then strain the petals through a sieve under running water.

The sugar, which you are going to use, can be pounded with the petals, to make the jam making process easier. That is how they used to do it in ancient times. You may also use crystallized sugar, but that is going to make it icky sweet.

The sugar amount is going to be exactly that much as the petals. So 2 cups of petals means 2 cups of sugar. But as I am making a number of bottles, I collect about 4 cups of petals.

When Is This Jam Normally Made

Gulkand is normally made in the summer. And it is going to be a slow cooking of the petals and the sugar in the sun in wide mouthed glass jars. Gulkand is definitely not made in plastic utensils. Sorry, it is also not made in earthenware pots. Come to think of it, why should not it be made in earthenware pots?

I guess all the moisture coming out from the sugar to make the jam is going to be absorbed in the earthenware pots. That seems to be a logical explanation. I wonder how the Empress Noor Jahan made her Gulkand –

glass or earthenware. She definitely did not use metal pots. Even though she had pots made of silver and gold, in which food was cooked specially for the impress of India. And she ate off silver platters.

Slow Sun Method

Now place the rose petals directly in the jars, in alternate layers. Alternating with the rose petals are going to be sugar layers. Do not fill the jar to the brim. Now, cover tightly and place out in the sun. The moisture is going to cook the jam into a jammy consistency.

Give the bottle a really good shake occasionally so that the jam gets a good chance to settle down well. Your long-lasting Gulkand is going to be cooked in 2 to 3 months, in the summer. Enjoy.

Fungal Infections in Nails

Have you noticed your nails getting disfigured because of fungal infections? These normally happen when you have been dabbling around in contaminated water or have been tiptoeing around the roses and daisies, bare feet.

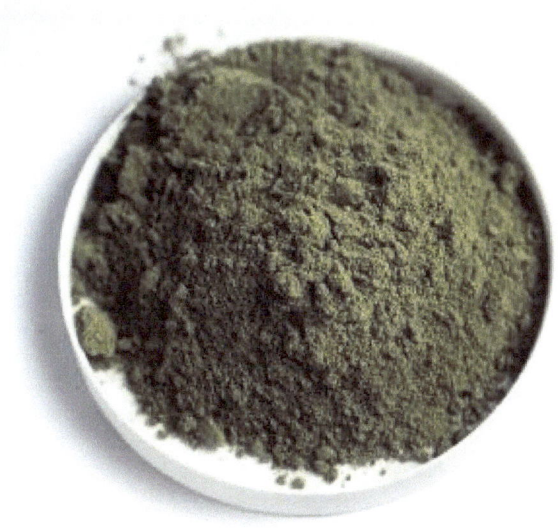

Powdered henna

This remedy was given to me by a person suffering from fungal infection on the palms of her hands. She wore henna designs on her hands, and that cured her! She told me that if people suffered from terrible fungal infections on their hands, or on their feet, fingers and toes, especially in the Nail area, all they had to do is dip that affected area in a paste of powdered henna – never mind the orange tint – once every day for a week, and see the infection clearing up miraculously.

This can only be done by people who do not mind their toes and nails being orange tinted but then that adornment can always be covered by closed shoes! So if you find fungus disfiguring your nails, just apply some paste of the henna with water, and allow to dry. It is going to take anywhere between 15 – 30 minutes for that paste to powder off in greenish brown flakes. It does not do you any harm, so you can leave it on with your orange tinted nails. Repeat this activity for the next week. Try not to walk in dirty, muddy water.

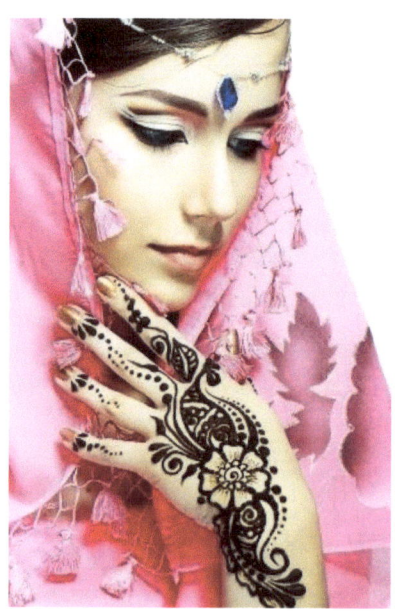

Eczema

You can also cure a case of eczema by making a mixture of five basil leaves and half a teaspoonful of lemon juice and applying it to the affected area. I normally used turpentine, because I did not know about this natural remedy. My job was to suffocate those parasites causing eczema. But now I can do the same with the basil and lemon cure.

The same positive results can also be obtained by applying lemon juice and garlic juice, if you do not have basil leaves around. Not bad! Renew this application, every day until you are totally cured.

Honey and Onion Mix

This is an extremely useful and easy cure for people suffering from nagging cough or even throat and chest congestion. Chop up an onion into pieces, put it in 3 tablespoons full of pure honey and leave it overnight. You are going to drink 1 tablespoon full of this onion honey three times a day, until your chest condition is cleared up. Try this right now.

You can also chop an onion in flakes and cover them with honey. Leave them in the shade for 3 hours. Keep drinking a teaspoonful of this resulting mixture throughout the day. You can also chew on the honeyed onion flakes.

Hiccup Cure

This is rather funny. This normally happens when something blocks your air passage, and you find yourself hiccupping and not even a glassful of water can unblock it. However, if you find it troubling you a lot, then it is not a state of amusement to you or your audience.

I remember once as a child, finding myself hiccupping away, and even putting my tongue out and panting and drinking water and swallowing salt could not manage to get rid of the hiccups.

So my grandmother had to resort to drastic measures, "Well then, I will have to tell your dad that somebody complained to me that you were stealing mangoes from their garden. They saw you. They are remembering you extremely angrily. That is why you cannot stop the hiccups.[1] "

I was totally flabbergasted and forgot my hiccups completely. So while protesting that I was innocent of such a calumny, and the person who said that was the biggest liar alive, I was cured.

So the answer is – grandma knows, the best way to scare someone into not hiccupping is to scare them out of their collective wits. This was also the

---

[1] This idea is very prevalent in the East. Hiccups are considered a sign that someone is trying to reach you desperately or is thinking of you. So one way in which we used to amuse ourselves at school, college and at office(!) – while hiccupping due to swallowing air with our refreshing drinks, – was to name all our acquaintances, according to the letters of the alphabet, saying, for example", R for Rita, is that you?" [hic!]. The idea was that when a person reached the right name, the hiccupping would stop. This will not work for a person with a very extensive social and enemy network!

first time I learned that Granny had an amazingly dry sense of humor and was not above using it when needed.

Anyway, this cure is equally drastic and effective. So if there is nobody human around to scare you, -nor can you find cockroaches or rats, rattlesnakes or lizards in the vicinity to help you forget your hiccupping,- just burn some freshly powdered peppercorns on the griddle, and inhale deeply. Naturally, you are going to start sneezing and that is going to clear up your passage.

Conclusion

I hope you found the information about grandma's natural remedies and ancient herbal recipes given in this book extremely useful. They are time-tested, so they are going to work. Nevertheless, some of these remedies take a little while, in order to help cure you. That is because some problems may be chronic, or your own health may prevent you from getting cured as fast as grandma could wish.

So stay healthy, keep healthy and look out for more grandma's natural remedies and ancient herbal recipes, which are going to keep you healthy and fit.

These books have food recipes, which help cure you. They also have ancient remedies which have been passed down the ages through generations, which have been keeping all those people healthy, when there were no experienced doctors around.

At that time. Grandma was more bothered about prevention is better than cure. That is why she made sure that her family ate healthy, stayed out in the open air, and came in a closed atmosphere, only at the end of the evening to sleep and eat. That is why the people of her generation and those of the generations before her were healthy. They believed in hard physical labor.

Unfortunately, there are only a few of us who still follow this lifestyle. We would rather sit in muggy, and ill ventilated rooms throughout the day, crouched in front of a computer or in front of the TV. We do not like exercising much. We also eat whatever comes at hand, because all of that is in plenty, and easily available, and it is tastier than healthy food.

No wonder our auto immune systems have deteriorated, and our naturally healthy genetic makeup is slowly and steadily growing weaker. That is why children of the next generation are prone to more genetic diseases, as well as diseases caused due to their surroundings.

So it is the time to look for healthy alternatives, in order to make you fit. It is only then you can raise a healthy and happy family. Naturally, you are going to be using purely natural products to help heal you.

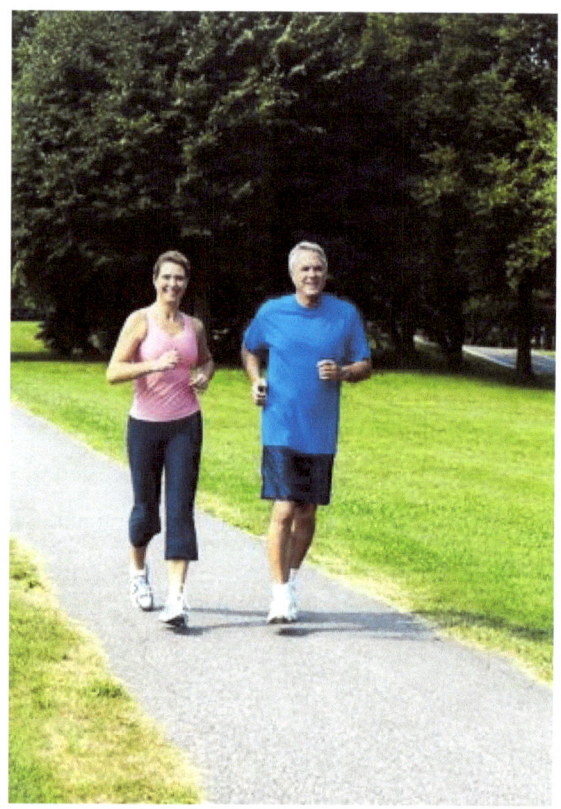

Life is for living and living emperor size! So eat healthy, live happy, live long, and prosper.

Appendix

Making Desi Ghee

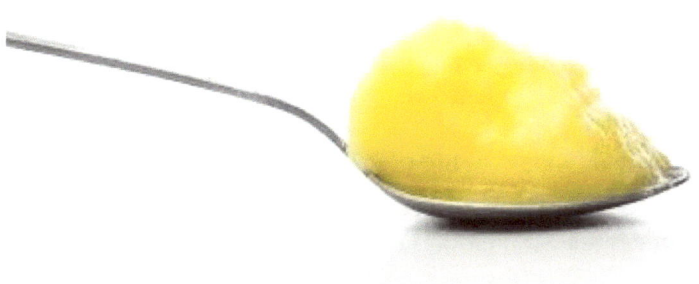

Pure Desi ghee is best made at home, because you are not going to be very sure about what you get in the market. It is often a mixture of other vegetable oils, with the percentage of Desi ghee being sold as pure clarified butter.

Desi ghee is clarified butter, which is extremely concentrated and a very powerful healing agent. It is normally used in the making up of herbal medicines, because it is made of pure creamy milk butter. It is also used in making beauty creams, potions, lotions and other skin ointments.

It has a powerful aroma, and that is why only just a spoonful is added to fry meats. It is going to float on the surface of the meat dish, after it has been cooked, so you need to stir the gravy before serving. Also, the food is not going to taste greasy, even though it looks like it has been swimming in fat.

Desi ghee is the concentrated form of pure butter, which is heated to reduce the butter of all the impurities as well as moisture. This concentrated butter is normally used in Eastern cuisine, for searing meat, sautéing and frying food, because they offer its higher burning point. You make this at home by taking 2 pounds of best unsalted butter and melting it in a heavy bottomed pan. Allow the butter to liquefy on low heat for about 40 minutes. Maintain this simmering point, until all of the moisture in the butter has evaporated. The impurities are going to sink to the bottom of the pan. Remember to keep stirring the butter, so that it does not burn.

Pour off the clear butter and strain it through several thicknesses of muslin cloth. This butter is going to last for about a year, if it is placed in a cool and dry place. This butter is exorbitantly expensive. So in the East, people with easy access to plenty fresh milk make it right in their kitchens for crisp delicious frying results, and adding that taste of pure butter to all their dishes.

Author Bio

Dueep Jyot Singh is a Management and IT Professional who managed to gather Postgraduate qualifications in Management and English and Degrees in Science, French and Education while pursuing different enjoyable career options like being an hospital administrator, IT,SEO and HRD Database Manager/ trainer, movie scriptwriter, theatre artiste and public speaker, lecturer in French, Marketing and Advertising, ex-Editor of Hearts On Fire (now known as Solstice) Books Missouri USA, advice columnist and cartoonist, publisher and Aviation School trainer, ex- moderator on Medico.in, banker, student councilor ,travelogue writer … among other things! One fine morning, she decided that she had enough of killing herself by Degrees and went back to her first love -- writing. It's more enjoyable! She already has 48 published academic and 14 fiction- in- different- genre books under her belt.

When she is not designing websites or making Graphic design illustrations for clients , she is browsing through old bookshops hunting for treasures, of which she has an enviable collection – including R.L. Stevenson, O.Henry, Dornford Yates, Maurice Walsh, C.N.Williamson, Sapper, Bartimeus and the crown of her collection- Dickens "The Old Curiosity Shop," and so on… Just call her "Renaissance Woman" - collecting herbal remedies, acting like Universal Helping Hand/Agony Aunt, or escaping to her dear mountains for a bit of exploring, collecting herbs and plants, and trekking.

Check out some of the other Health Learning Series books at Amazon.com

Health Learning Series on Amazon

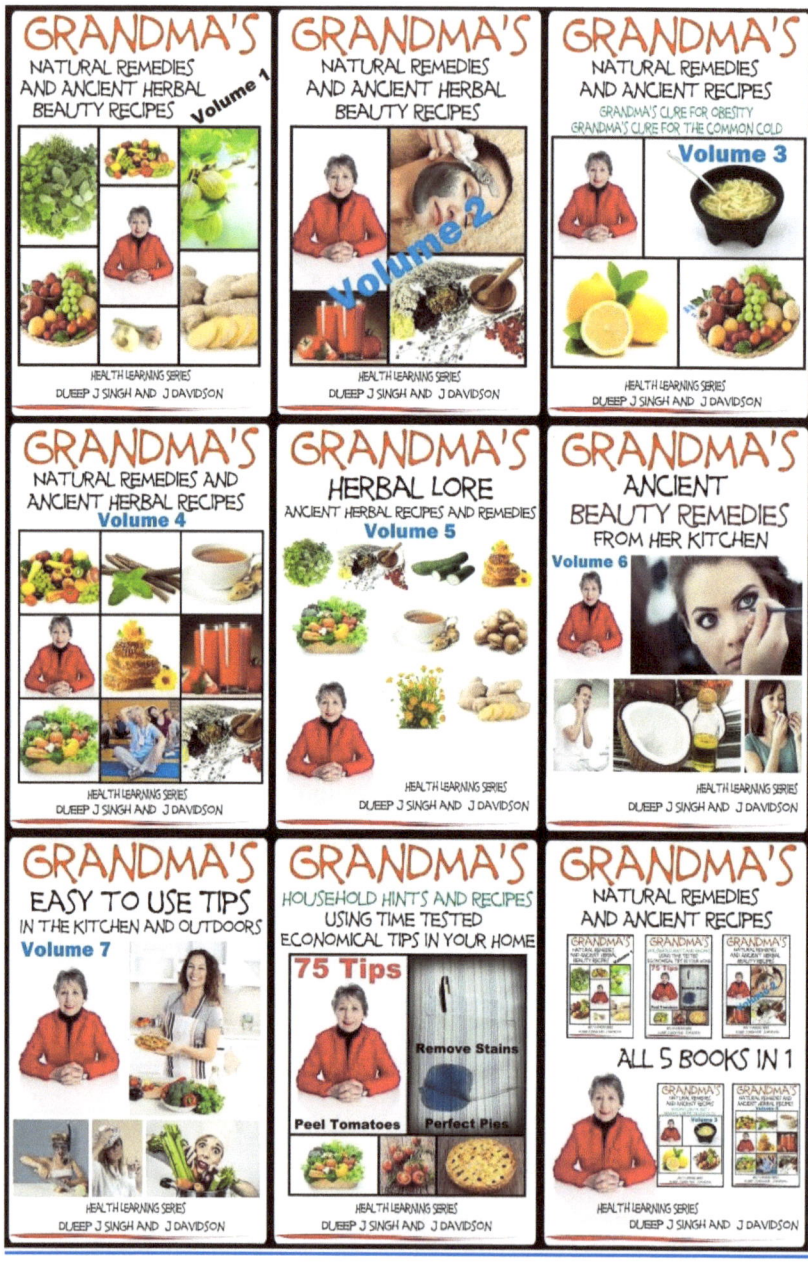

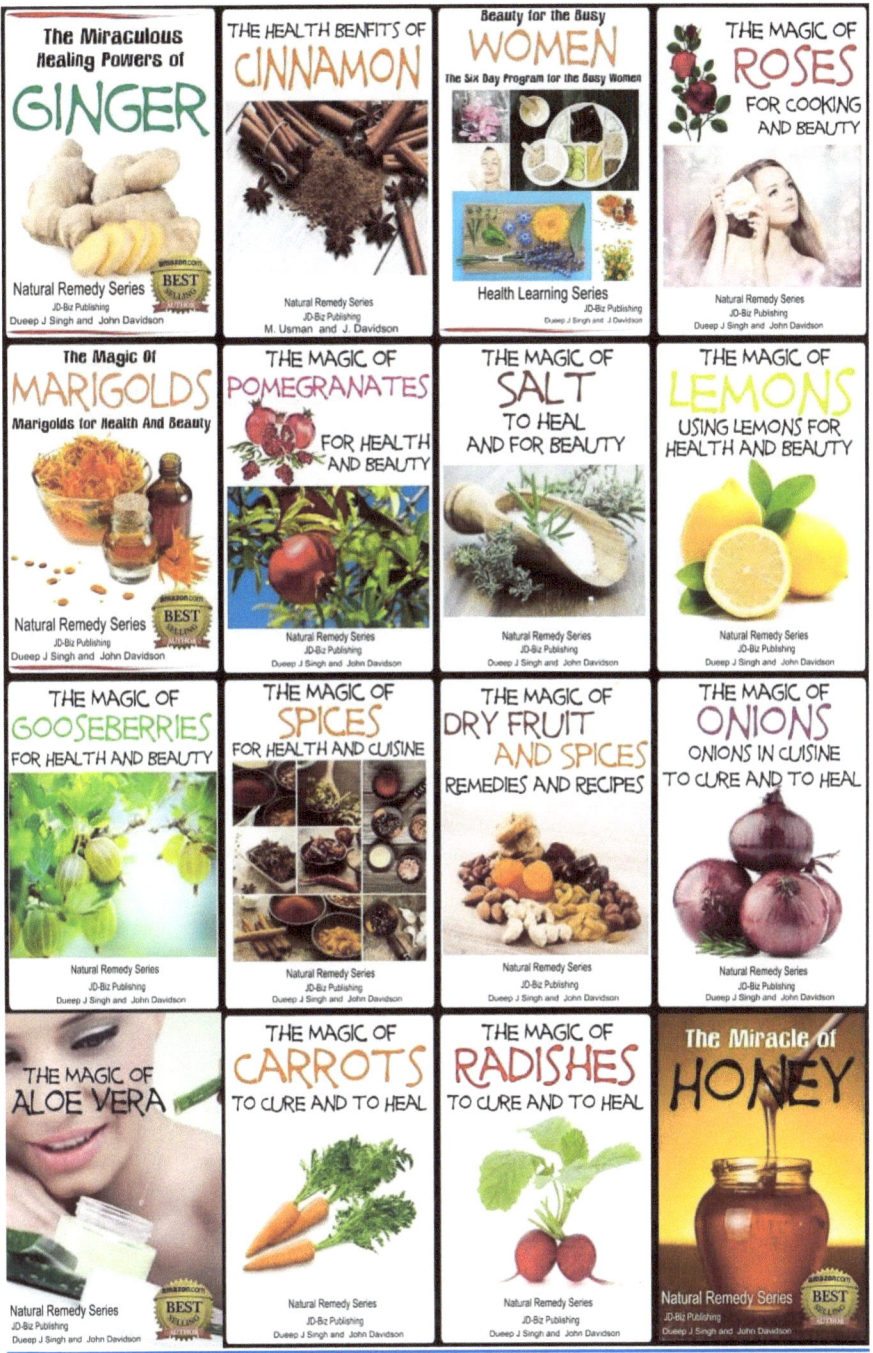

The Miraculous Healing Powers of GINGER
Natural Remedy Series
JD-Biz Publishing
Dueep J Singh and John Davidson

THE HEALTH BENFITS OF CINNAMON
Natural Remedy Series
JD-Biz Publishing
M. Usman and J. Davidson

Beauty for the Busy WOMEN
The Six Day Program for the Busy Women
Health Learning Series
JD-Biz Publishing
Dueep J Singh and J Davidson

THE MAGIC OF ROSES
FOR COOKING AND BEAUTY
Natural Remedy Series
JD-Biz Publishing
Dueep J Singh and John Davidson

The Magic Of MARIGOLDS
Marigolds for Health And Beauty
Natural Remedy Series
JD-Biz Publishing
Dueep J Singh and John Davidson

THE MAGIC OF POMEGRANATES
FOR HEALTH AND BEAUTY
Natural Remedy Series
JD-Biz Publishing
Dueep J Singh and John Davidson

THE MAGIC OF SALT
TO HEAL AND FOR BEAUTY
Natural Remedy Series
JD-Biz Publishing
Dueep J Singh and John Davidson

THE MAGIC OF LEMONS
USING LEMONS FOR HEALTH AND BEAUTY
Natural Remedy Series
JD-Biz Publishing
Dueep J Singh and John Davidson

THE MAGIC OF GOOSEBERRIES
FOR HEALTH AND BEAUTY
Natural Remedy Series
JD-Biz Publishing
Dueep J Singh and John Davidson

THE MAGIC OF SPICES
FOR HEALTH AND CUISINE
Natural Remedy Series
JD-Biz Publishing
Dueep J Singh and John Davidson

THE MAGIC OF DRY FRUIT AND SPICES
REMEDIES AND RECIPES
Natural Remedy Series
JD-Biz Publishing
Dueep J Singh and John Davidson

THE MAGIC OF ONIONS
ONIONS IN CUISINE TO CURE AND TO HEAL
Natural Remedy Series
JD-Biz Publishing
Dueep J Singh and John Davidson

THE MAGIC OF ALOE VERA
Natural Remedy Series
JD-Biz Publishing
Dueep J Singh and John Davidson

THE MAGIC OF CARROTS
TO CURE AND TO HEAL
Natural Remedy Series
JD-Biz Publishing
Dueep J Singh and John Davidson

THE MAGIC OF RADISHES
TO CURE AND TO HEAL
Natural Remedy Series
JD-Biz Publishing
Dueep J Singh and John Davidson

The Miracle of HONEY
Natural Remedy Series
JD-Biz Publishing
Dueep J Singh and John Davidson

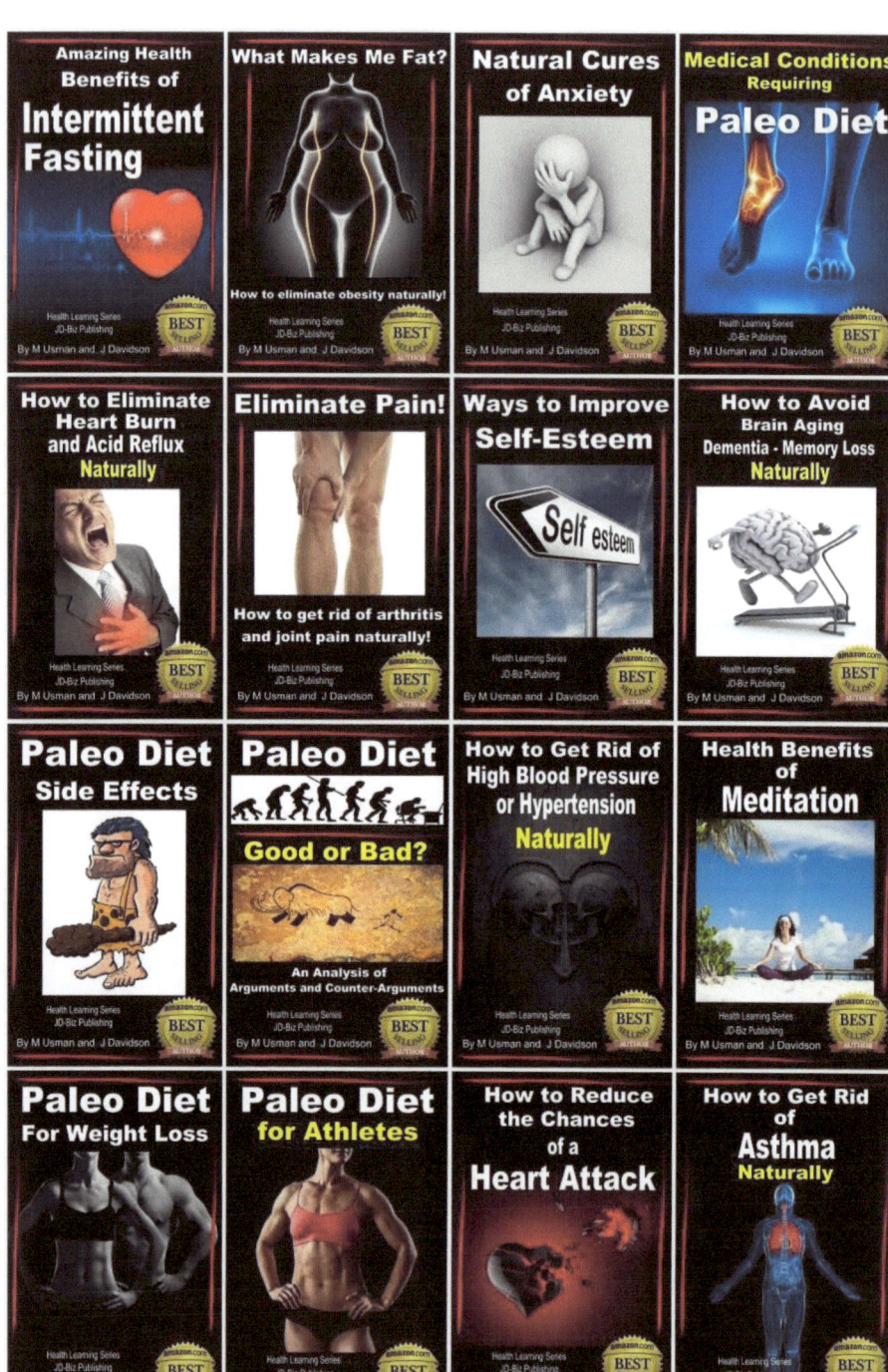

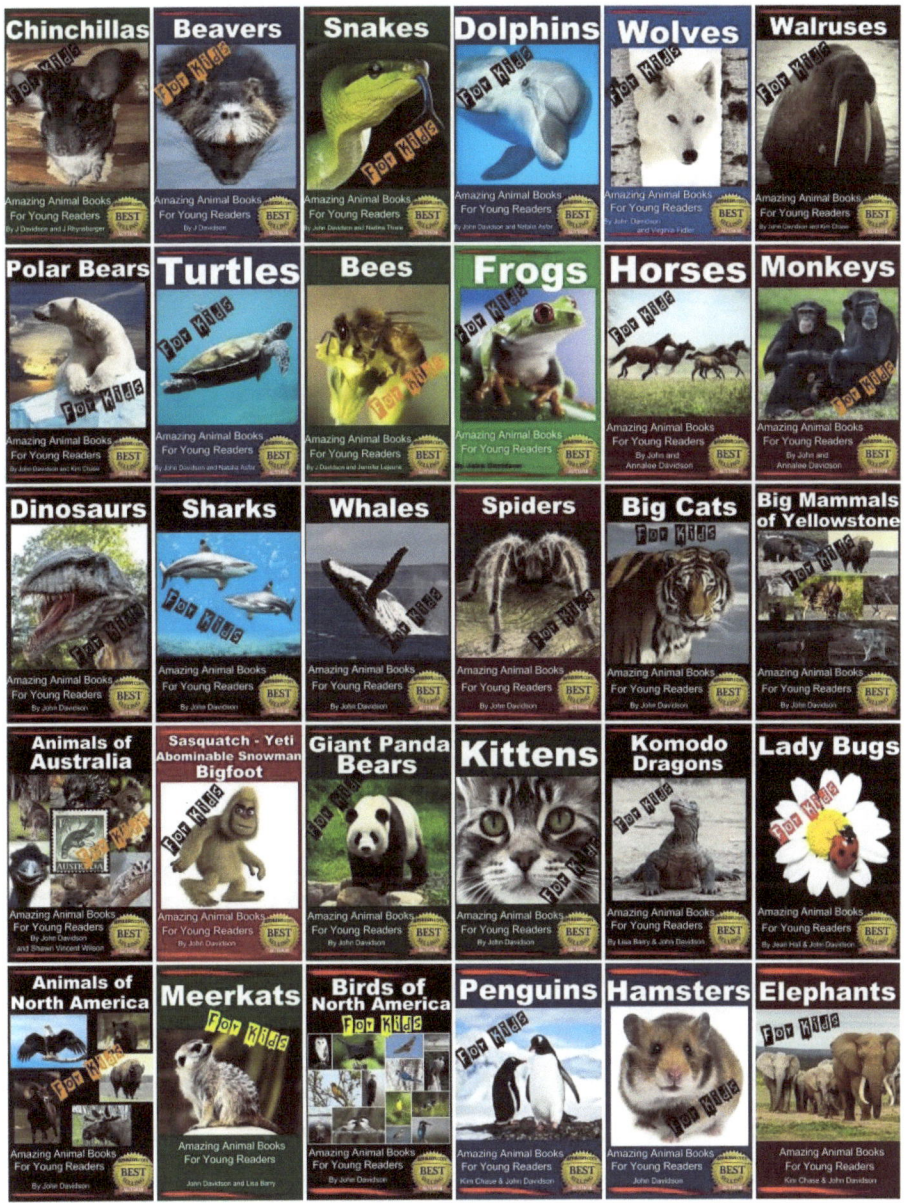

Learn To Draw Series

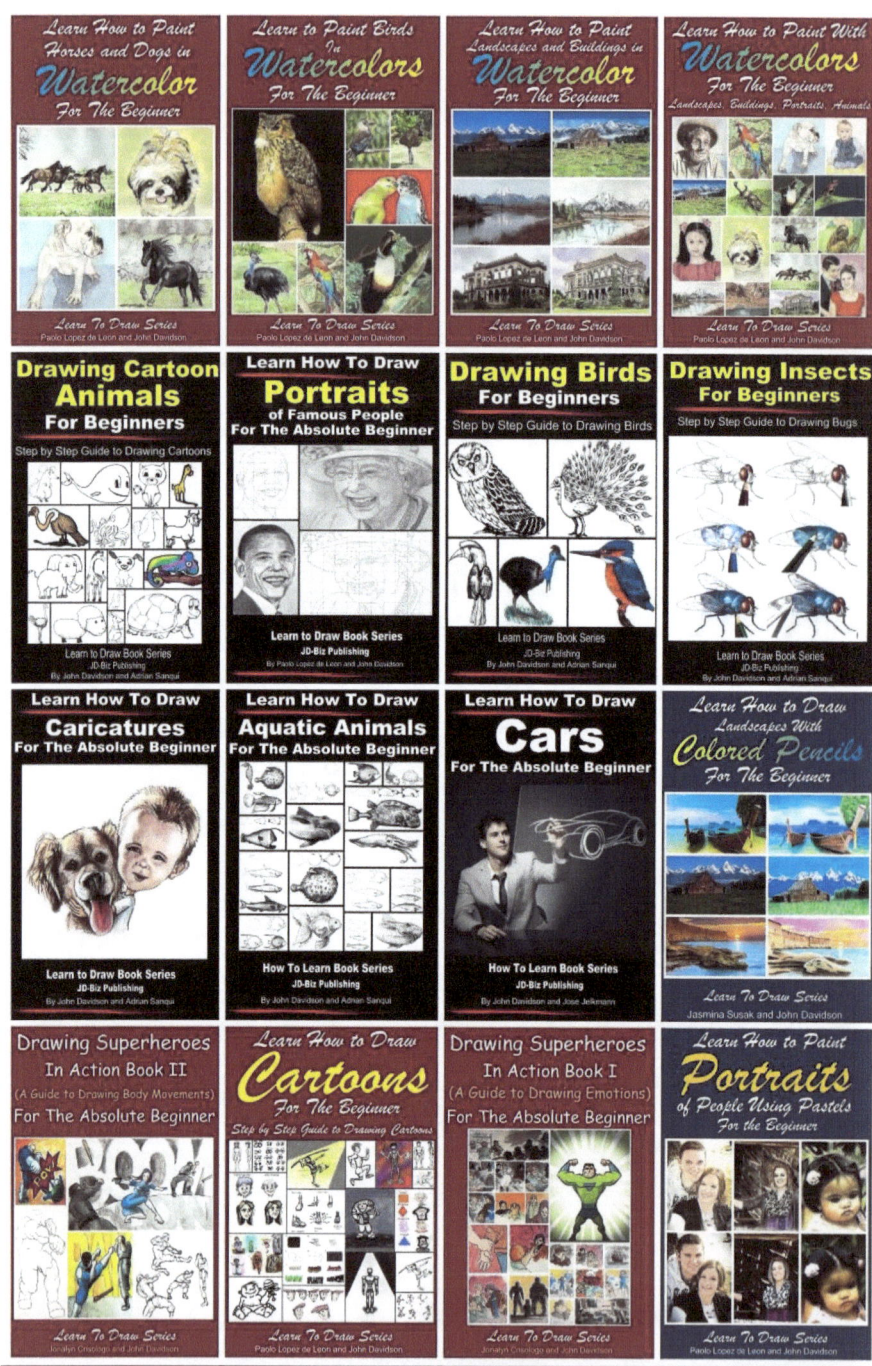

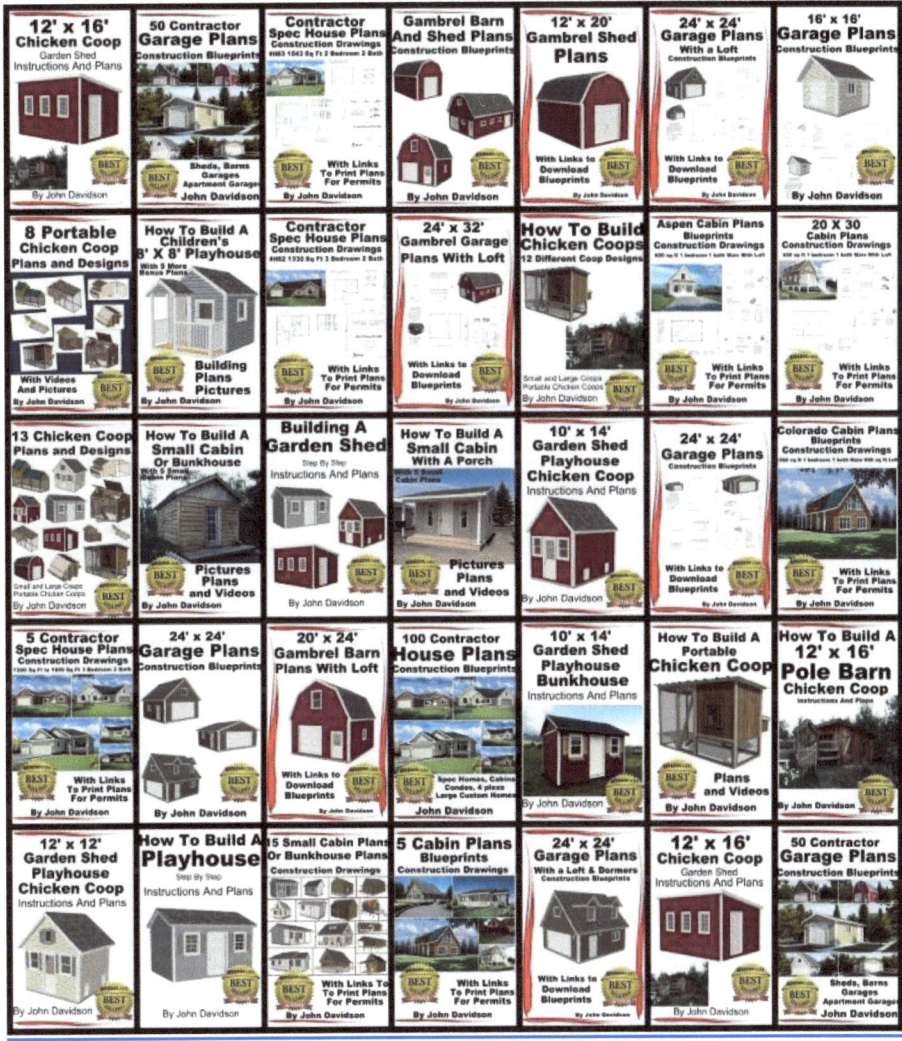

Our books are available at

1. Amazon.com

2. Barnes and Noble

3. Itunes

4. Kobo

5. Smashwords

6. Google Play Books

Download Free Books!

http://MendonCottageBooks.com

Publisher

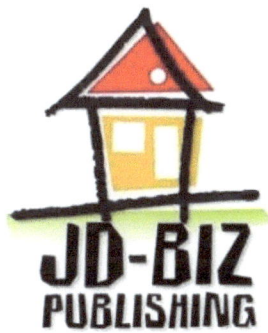

JD-Biz Corp

P O Box 374

Mendon, Utah 84325

http://www.jd-biz.com/

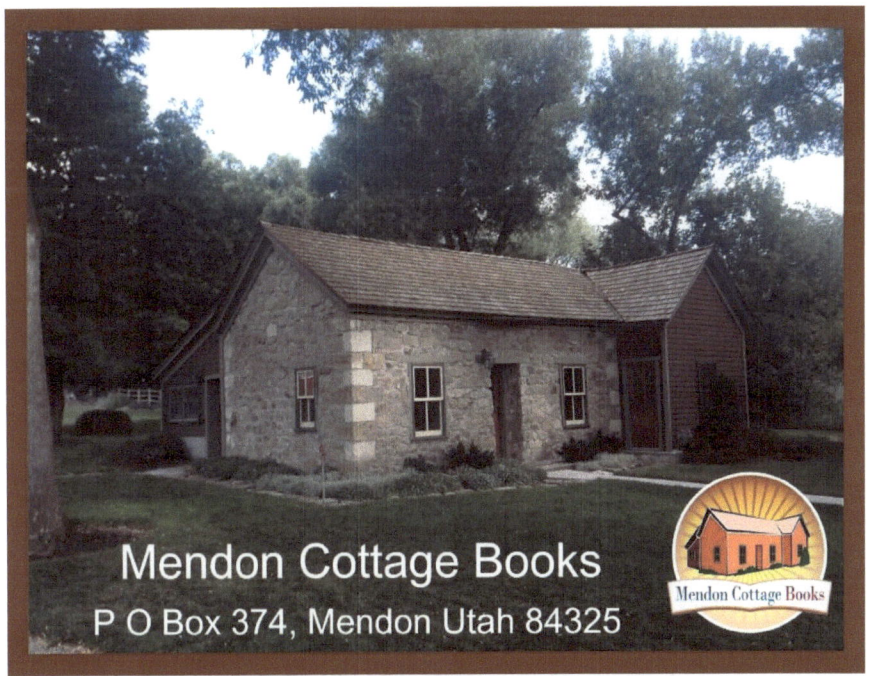

www.ingramcontent.com/pod-product-compliance
Lightning Source LLC
Chambersburg PA
CBHW050837290526
45792CB00001B/429